THE DOC̄ ̄ ̄
PRES̲

*Prevention

MW00440900

By
Kenneth Wright
in consultation with
In consultation with the WOCN (Wound Ostomy Continence Nurses)
association, The AHCPR (Agency for Health Care Policy and Research),
the NPUAP (National Pressure Advisory Ulcer Advisory Panel).
Our special thanks for the editing and contributions from Dr. Shamil
Kumar, Dr. W. Jensen, Sharlene Wiley BSN, CETN, Heather Orsted,
M.Sc., RN, BN, ET, Rick Fontaine and all the nurses that completed the
editorial survey from the WOCN and CAWC.
The content of this book adheres to the recognized best practice
guidelines from the various authoritative North American associations
and have been adapted for the lay reader.

ISBN # 1 55040 -830-5
Pressure Ulcers. Pressure sores. Self-help. Decubitus ulcers. Skin ulcers.
Wound care.

©2005, 2006, 2007, 2008, 2009, 2010, 2016 Mediscript Communications
Inc.
E mail mediscript30@yahoo.ca, Tel 800 773 5088, fax 800 639 3186

www.mediscript.net

MEDISCRIPT HEALTH EDUCATION SERVICES

Making information work for you

Doctor Guide Books
For patient counseling & compliance

Easy to read like Readers" Digest
Saves you time
Nothing controversial –mainstream
Generic information on treatments
Self help preventative tips

Training workshops for health workers
CDslides,facilitatornotes,delegatemanual

Ensure quality assurance standard
Economical – cost effective
Retain & motivate staff
Increased performance
Comply with accreditation guidelines

TITLES

Pressure Ulcers
Venous Leg Ulcer
Incontinence care
Diabetic Foot Ulcers
Diabetes and Feet
Urostomies
Ileostomies
Colostomies
How to Stop Smoking
COPD prevention & treatment

PROGRAMS

Alzheimer's Disease
Type 2 Diabetes
Stroke
Brain Injury
Multiple Sclerosis
Arthritis
Pain in the older client
Nutrition & Aging
Preventing Falls
Elder abuse

For full listing go to www.mediscript.net
Tel: 800 773 5088 • Fax 800 639 3186 • email: medicript30@yahoo.ca

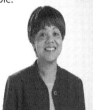
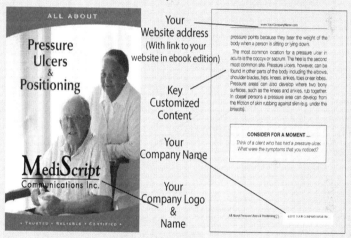
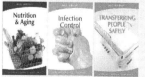

Table of Contents

Continued on next page

SECTION 3:
PRESSURE ULCER TREATMENT

SECTION 4: APPENDIX

IMPORTANT MESSAGE FROM THE PUBLISHER

A note of caution

This book provides generic information in harmony with the "best practices guidelines" documented by expert organizations. See appendix for web sites.

However treatment and advice on preventing and caring for pressure ulcers are wide – ranging and depend upon the health care practitioner's diagnosis and assessment of the patient's condition. Consequently this book is not a substitute for the health care practitioner's advice and treatment. With this in mind the publisher and authors disclaim any responsibility for any adverse effects resulting directly or indirectly from suggestions, undetected errors or from misunderstanding on the part of the reader.

The reader

The book is appropriate for many health care workers known as the following (depending upon geographic region or type of work):

Personal Support Worker, Unlicensed Care Provider, Home Support Worker, Home Care Aides, Nurse Aides, Nursing Assistants, Personal Care Attendants, Unlicensed Assistive Personnel, Community Health Workers. The book is also appropriate for caregivers, family members of patients or patients.

Ordering more copies

Thanks to sponsorship, this book is available at discounted prices for as low as $1.50 depending upon quantity.

Other appropriate titles are available such as Venous Leg Ulcers, Incontinence Care, Diabetic Foot Ulcers, Urostomy Care… etc.

visit www.mediscript.net to review full range of titles.

email: mediscript30@yahoo.ca.

Telephone: 800 773 5088 • Fax: 800 639 3186.

Notes

Section 1
Understanding

INTRODUCTION

In order to understand what we're dealing with, let's take a look at the title of this book. Pressure ulcers have been given many names – bedsores, skin ulcers, wounds, decubitus ulcers – but they all mean essentially the same thing. The important thing to understand is that the information in this book can help all these conditions.

WHO SHOULD BE READING THIS BOOK?

- You are a health care worker, care provider or support staff, and you want a comprehensive, easy to understand reference guide on all the issues.
- You are a health care professional and you want to help your patients understand and prevent pressure ulcers, or help in the healing process of existing pressure ulcers.
- Someone in your family has a pressure ulcer problem and you want to help.
- You are at risk of developing a pressure ulcer and you want to prevent it from happening.

BENEFITS OF READING THIS BOOK

- You will understand why a person can be at risk of developing pressure ulcers.
- You can actually prevent a pressure ulcer from occurring.
- You can avoid costly treatments by taking preventive action when the first signs of a pressure ulcer become evident.
- You can speed the healing process of the pressure ulcer.

Notes

PREVENTION AND TREATMENT IS A TEAM EFFORT

The support worker or care - provider are the front line health workers, caring directly for patients, who are pivotal to the success of the prevention and treatment activities. There are also many other health professionals who are involved, such as, home care nurses, dietitians, family physicians and others.

It must be realized that this is a team effort and everybody should be working from the "same page". Hopefully this book will provide the uniformity of information for the whole team, perhaps just basic information for the health care professionals but perhaps a little technical for the patient. With this in mind this book can be the catalyst for discussion and understanding.

PATIENT POWER

How a person copes with a pressure ulcer or the threat of one developing can contribute significantly to a successful outcome. The nurse, support worker, care – provider and other members of the team all need the cooperation of the patient if the pressure ulcer is to be prevented or healed. Consequently taking an holistic approach of treating the whole patient with their involvement in care practices is very important.

FINAL NOTE

Some diseases have a predictable outcome over time and there is little you can do except to try to improve the patient's quality of life. Pressure ulcers, however, can be prevented and healing can be speeded up by following the instructions of the health care professional. So, when it comes to avoiding a pressure ulcer, prevention is the order of the day.

The major contributing factor of pressure ulcers is unequalized pressure creating an inadequate blood supply (known as ischemia) to the "at risk" skin area. However, there are many factors that, along with pressure, contribute to the formation of an ulcer. It is important to recognize the individuality of each case and, because of this, we have provided opportunities throughout this book to write down specific advice and treatment guidelines. Be sure to do this, and refer to your notes regularly.

PREVENTION IS BETTER THAN CURE

Current statistics show that each year in North America well over 1,000,000 people who are receiving care in hospitals, nursing homes or at home, develop pressure ulcers. It is estimated that the cost of treating a pressure ulcer can exceed $40,000 so in strictly financial terms it makes great sense to prevent the condition.

Pressure ulcers are often called bedsores because they are most common to people who are confined to their beds. However, anybody can develop these painful skin problems.

Essentially, pressure ulcers occur when any part of a person's body is kept in one position for too long. Healthy people naturally move about and change position so that these ulcers do not develop. Consequently, the types of patients who are at risk include people with joint disorders, plaster casts or paralysis, those who are unconscious and those who are in wheel chairs. In fact, anybody who is immobile is at risk of developing this condition and it is common for a hospital patient to have his or her hospital stay prolonged because of the development of these ulcers.

Pressure ulcers can be painful, ugly and downright depressing. Let this book help you to prevent them in the first place, and provide a better quality of life for your client, yourself or a loved one.

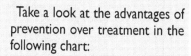

Take a look at the advantages of prevention over treatment in the following chart:

Notes

Prevention Versus Treatment

Prevention Method	Treatment Method
Little effort needed.	Demanding for both patient and caregiver.
Patient comfort assured.	Possible patient stress, discomfort and pain.
Patient in control.	Patient dependent upon medical staff.
Not expensive.	Costly due to medications, dressings, laundry, medical staff, etc.
Medical staff less involved—perhaps in advisory capacity.	Medical staff actively involved.
No presciptions necessary.	Prescibed medications sometimes needed.
Safe procedures.	Risk of complications.
Reduces hospital stay.	Can increase time of hospitalization.
Post hospitalization seldom required.	Continued post hospitalization services, medical appointments necessary.
No recurrence possible.	Recurrence possible.

Everybody's Different

The mix of preventive measures and treatment for a pressure ulcer is specific to each person, but there are general guidelines that are important to understand. Indeed, the most important goal of this book is to provide understanding of the nature of a pressure ulcer so that the actions you take make sense and motivate you to comply with your health care professional's directions.

Once you understand the causes of a pressure ulcer and the nature of the problem, all your actions will appear to be common sense and you will be able to take the initiative in speeding up the healing process. Once you are comfortable with the information presented in this book, makes notes, develop specific prevention measures and try to make these measures become habits for all involved from the patient to the support worker, care provider, caregiver and all members of the health care team.

WHAT IS A PRESSURE ULCER?

Put simply, a pressure ulcer usually appears as an open wound due to the skin becoming so badly damaged that it breaks down or dies. The problem can present itself as a simple nuisance or as a life-threatening condition.

A number of factors can contribute to the development of a pressure ulcer but the cause is unequalized pressure (usually in bony areas such as the heel of the foot, the elbow, the lower back or the shoulders) for an extended period of time because the patient is inactive, confined perhaps to a bed or wheelchair. Although further details will be given later, the simple reason for the pressure is the reduced blood supply to the area.

In its early stages, a pressure ulcer can appear harmless enough – the color of the skin turns pink or red and does not return to normal after the pressure is removed. As the condition worsens, the skin eventually becomes cracked, blistered or broken.

In order to better understand the concept, consider what happens when a tourniquet is applied to a badly bleeding wound to reduce the blood supply and prevent massive bleeding. Pressure on the skin and underlying tissue works like a tourniquet in that

Notes

it prevents the supply of blood and nutrients from reaching that particular area. If the situation becomes chronic, cells will die. In fact, once the skin color turns from red or pink to white, and remains white, deterioration of the skin and tissue has already occurred.

Earlier we mentioned that there are other names for pressure ulcers, so let's get the terminology into perspective. Keep in mind that the cause and basic treatment principles are the same for all of these conditions. The name difference is related to the possible cause of the ulcer, the preference of the health care practitioner and the area of skin at risk.

Pressure Ulcer

In medical terms, an ulcer refers to a crater-like lesion. A peptic ulcer, for instance, has the same characteristics but is found in the stomach and is caused by distinctive factors that differ from those which cause pressure ulcers.

Bed Sore

Skin breakdown often happens to people who are bedridden and not very mobile. Continuous unequalized pressure is exerted on certain parts of the body due to lack of movement. The condition can be tender and painful.

Decubitus Ulcer

This is the traditional medical term. Decubitus (pronounced dee-CUBE-i-tus) derives from the Latin word "decumbere" meaning to lie down, referring to its frequent occurrence among people who are immobile and confined to bed.

Leg Ulcer

The leg ulcer differs from other types of skin wounds because of its unique causative factors and requires a more complicated treatment plan, which we will not go into here.

Wound

A wound is a break in the skin, usually associated with physical injury. This is possibly the furthest removed term for a pressure ulcer but the medical profession often includes this term in the pressure ulcer category. It's fair to note that a normal wound, with none of the high-risk factors such as poor circulation, or pressure on the skin due to immobility, will generally heal more quickly than a pressure ulcer.

Whenever you hear any of these terms – with the possible exception of wound – you can be assured that they mean the same thing as a pressure ulcer. Although we have decided to use the term pressure ulcer throughout this book, don't be confused if your nurse, health care professional or physician calls your condition by any of the other names we have listed. As we said earlier, it's often simply a matter of personal preference.

Notes

WHAT CAUSES A PRESSURE ULCER?

In order to understand how pressure ulcers occur, it helps if you understand the nature and interaction of your skin and circulatory system.

SKIN

Just like your heart, liver or kidney, your skin is an organ of your body. The major function of your skin is to act like a wrapper or package to contain your skeleton and other organs. Essentially, your skin has a protective function and is inherently strong, pliable and elastic – the ideal characteristics for a "wrapping" function.

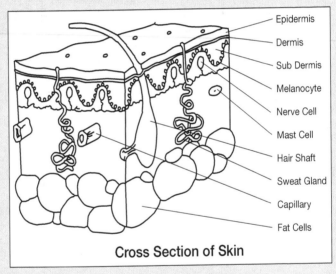

Epidermis
Dermis
Sub Dermis
Melanocyte
Nerve Cell
Mast Cell
Hair Shaft
Sweat Gland
Capillary
Fat Cells

Cross Section of Skin

THE CIRCULATORY SYSTEM

We all know about arteries and veins, the vessels that form a network of rivers carrying blood, pumped by the heart, to every part of your body. In simple terms, your arteries transport oxygenated blood. Veins return deoxygenated blood (blood with the oxygen replaced by carbon dioxide) back to your heart for circulation through your lungs where the oxygen is replenished.

Notes

We are now going to ask you to get out an imaginary microscope and examine your circulatory system on a much smaller scale. Our bodies are made up of billions of individual cells. These living cells are bathed in a sea of fluids which contain oxygen, nutrients, hormones and wastes. The rivers of blood flow through this sea nourishing, cleansing and chemically balancing it.

The arteries themselves break down into much smaller vessels, called capillaries, which are one cell thick and highly permeable. This allows for the vital, life-giving exchange to take place between the rivers and the sea of intracellular fluids.

To continue our analogy, the capillaries can be compared to a barge moored alongside a quay where cargoes are swapped. In this case, the cargoes are oxygen, carbon dioxide, nutrients, waste products, hormones and minerals.

One third of our bodies' blood supply flows through our skin. The blood nourishes the cells of the skin and removes waste, ensuring that our skin remains healthy and functional.

SKIN + CIRCULATORY SYSTEM + PROBLEMS = PRESSURE ULCERS

Put in simple terms, a pressure ulcer can develop because of reduced blood flow or because the "integrity" of the skin has been damaged.

It's important to understand all the possible factors that contribute to creating a pressure ulcer. We have already highlighted the most common, and therefore most important problem – unequalized pressure on the skin – which we will now explain in more detail.

PRIMARY CAUSE OF PRESSURE ULCERS:
Unequalized Pressure

Unequalized pressure is caused by the weight of the body pressing the skin against a surface hard enough to slow or stop the flow of blood in the area. If the surface is hard and particularly if unequalized pressure occurs over a bony, thin-skinned area, there is a definite risk of a pressure ulcer developing.

The subsequent reduced blood flow to the skin inhibits vital nourishment from the blood; consequently, the skin becomes damaged and breaks down or dies, leaving an open wound.

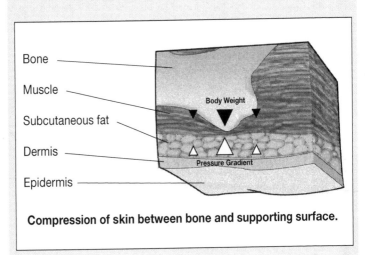

Bone
Muscle
Subcutaneous fat
Dermis
Epidermis

Body Weight

Pressure Gradient

Compression of skin between bone and supporting surface.

Pressure ulcers occur this way most commonly where the skin is thinnest, over a bony area such as the heels, lower back, elbows or shoulders. When the patient becomes immobilized and body movements are restricted, the weight of the body no longer has an opportunity to shift from one position to another, as it will normally do even in sleep. The soft tissue or skin trapped between the bed and the bony prominences is compressed under the weight of the body and capillary blood flow is reduced or completely cut off.

The following illustrations depict the areas of the body which are most at risk in various situations:

PRESSURE POINTS

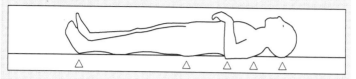
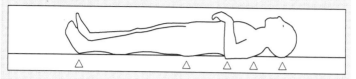

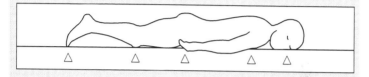

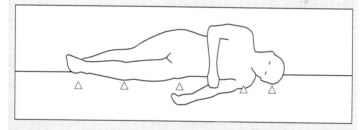

Common pressure points

One must be aware that the threshold or point of breakdown will vary considerably from patient to patient. For one person, damage may occur after only an hour or two of extended unequalized pressure, while another individual may be more fortunate. Because of this, it is important to inspect the skin frequently in order to determine the susceptibility and risk areas for any particular patient.

We cannot overstate the importance of this point: unequalized pressure on the skin is the primary cause of pressure ulcers. Careful planning in order to reduce the possibility of these ulcers occurring is perhaps the most important contribution you can make!

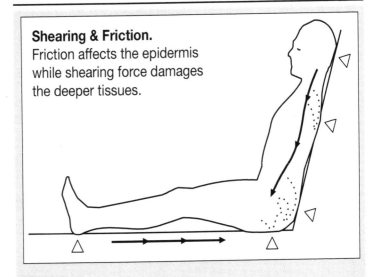

Shearing & Friction.
Friction affects the epidermis
while shearing force damages
the deeper tissues.

OTHER CAUSES OF PRESSURE ULCERS
Shearing force
A person confined to a bed sliding slowly downwards from the sitting position best exemplifies this. The consequent pulling or stretching of the skin can interrupt the blood supply to the skin.

Friction
Friction can be created when skin and sheets or bedclothes rub together. This may happen when:
- A person is pulled across rough or wrinkled sheets.
- Food crumbs have not been removed.
- Skin rubs against a body brace or traction device.

Skin exposure to moisture
Constant skin exposure to moisture through incontinence (leaking urine), perspiration or wound drainage can contribute to rashes, chafing, cracking of the skin or infection. The two most important preventative actions to avoid skin breakdown is a) the use of absorbent disposable incontinence products that have the ability to absorb moisture and provide a quick drying interface and b) using skin moisture protectant products.

Perspiration

This is most often caused by inappropriate bedding, fever, garments and so on. Perspiration moisture contributes to skin breakdown through chafing and cracking of the skin.

Unhealthy skin

Disease, old age, poor circulation, skin dryness, lack of exercise, the use of irritating creams or ointments and improper humidity and temperature are all factors in contributing to unhealthy skin. Some of these are out of your hands and only medical treatment can help, but there are some things you can do. (We'll go into more detail about this later in the section on skin care.)

Poor nutrition

General health and good skin integrity often depend on good eating habits. There can be many simple reasons why a person is not eating properly. Inappropriate plates and utensils, for example, or unappealing meals or a despondent attitude – these can all be factors. If a pressure ulcer already exists, proper nutrition becomes even more critical.

Poor hygiene

A lack of planning or motivation, inappropriate undergarments, inconvenient facilities – the list of factors contributing to poor hygiene can be long. Although it does require some effort, proper hygiene is one factor that can be controlled.

Old age

Let's not forget the obvious: with aging, major changes occur in the skin. For one thing, the amount of fat on the legs and forearms is usually reduced, cutting down on valuable padding and predisposing elderly patients to pressure ulcers. This is also why older people are more likely to complain of being cold. As we age, our sweat glands diminish in number, causing dry, itchy skin.

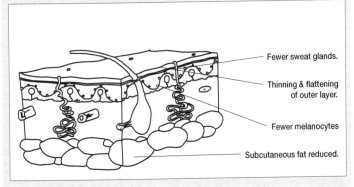

Notes

Effects of aging on skin

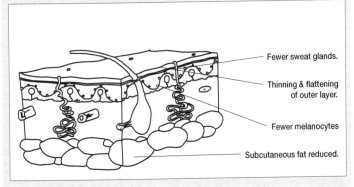

Fewer sweat glands.

Thinning & flattening of outer layer.

Fewer melanocytes

Subcutaneous fat reduced.

Shrinkage of collagen and elastic fibers causes thin, inelastic skin, and weakening of the attachment between the dermis and epidermis. This may result in minor friction or shearing forces to cause the skin layers to separate, or tear.

While all of the above factors are the most important elements in contributing to the problem, there are other situations which can potentially pose a threat.

They are:

Obesity:
This can cause increased pressure on the skin.

Emaciation:
Extreme body thinness leaving less protection over the bones.

Edema:
Swelling of tissues affecting blood flow.

Anemia:
A lack of nutrients affects the quality of the blood supply to the skin.

Mental confusion or apathy:
This can affect self-care habits.

Any one of these factors or a combination of several of them can cause a pressure ulcer to develop. As the major focus should be on preventing the development of pressure ulcers as opposed to treating them once they occur, the next logical step should be to identify who is at risk of developing a pressure ulcer. This will enable you to translate the causes of pressure ulcers into patient profiles.

WHO IS AT RISK?

If you are a caregiver, this section is extremely important. An understanding of the causes of pressure ulcers linked with the patient's characteristics can provide you with the tools to prevent a great deal of suffering and medical costs. When you can predict you can often prevent!

We now know that the primary cause of a pressure ulcer is unequalized pressure on the skin for extended periods of time.
Consequently, the most significant risk factor is inactivity and immobility. Anyone who is unable to move is in danger.
These factors are also often linked to a person's mental state. An individual who is lethargic, confused, semi-comatose or completely unconscious is a high-risk patient.

The highest risk categories for developing pressure ulcers are:
•Spinal cord injuries
•Bedridden patients
•Unconscious patients
•Severe or chronic injuries
•Post surgical patients (temporarily at high risk)
•Patients with contractures
•Incontinent patients

Notes

As you can appreciate, pressure ulcers know no boundaries – young and old, male and female are all potential victims.

If you wish to pursue this further, the Pressure Ulcer Risk Calculator on the following page is a simple and objective way to determine the extent to which a patient is at risk of developing a pressure ulcer.

Several clinical conditions are assessed and given a score. If the total score amounts to 14 or less, the patient should be considered at risk of developing pressure ulcers. It will then become necessary to take preventive measures.

You now have objective information to determine whether the person in your care is at risk of developing pressure ulcers. This can be a very useful guide and should motivate you to inspect the skin in the body areas prone to developing pressure ulcers. The next critical skill you must develop is the ability to effectively inspect the skin and to know what to look for. Read Stage I and Stage II on page 23.

The opposite "Risk Calculator" is a simple adaption from the more comprehensive and detailed "Braden Scale for Predicting Pressure Sore Risk ®. For interested readers and health care professionals the complete scale can be found at www.bradenscale.com

This site will provide the specific parameters with qualifying remarks to provide a more detailed assessment and recommended treatments for a particular pressure ulcer.

PRESSURE ULCER RISK CALCULATOR

Directions: Choose the appropriate numbers from the rating scale and add them up. The lower the score, the greater the risk. A score of 14 or less indicates the patient is at risk. (Adapted with permission from the Braden Scale for Predicting Pressure Sore Risk®.)

Physical condition	Rating	Score
Good	4	
Fair	3	
Poor	2	
Very bad	1	
Mental condition	**Rating**	**Score**
Alert	4	
Apathetic	3	
Confused	2	
Stuporous	1	
Activity	**Rating**	**Score**
Ambulant	4	
Walks with help	3	
Chairbound	2	
Bedfast	1	
Mobility	**Rating**	**Score**
Full	4	
Slightly	3	
Very limited	2	
None	1	
Incontinence	**Rating**	**Score**
None	4	
Occasional	3	
Usual/urine	2	
Double	1	
Total Score		

A low score in *any* category should initiate "intervention" to improve that risk factor. For example, a rating of 2 (Very limited) for Mobility suggests physical therapy, passive therapy or range of motion at the bedside should be implemented.

Notes

HOW TO RECOGNIZE A
PRESSURE ULCER

Once a pressure ulcer has developed, it can rapidly get worse unless you take quick action to treat it. Again, we must emphasize the importance of contacting a doctor or nurse to attend to it in the early stages, thereby avoiding more extensive treatment and the accompanying costs and inconvenience.

The first two stages are the most significant in obtaining a quick reversal and normal health. However, a discussion of the final two stages may help you to understand the potential severity of the condition and appreciate the critical importance of preventive procedures.

The following section will describe the four classical stages of a pressure ulcer. With proper care, the first two stages can take a short time to heal. As soon as you notice a skin problem, contact the doctor or nurse immediately and follow the instructions given to you exactly.

The following pages of classifying the four stages Pressure Ulcers was accurately developed by the National Pressure Ulcer Advisory Panel (NPUAP) and further information for the health care professional or interested reader can be found at www.npuap.org

STAGE I
Description and Symptoms

This is the mild stage, appearing as pink, red, or mottled, unbroken skin that stays that way for more than 20 minutes after the pressure is relieved (an African-American person's skin may look purple.) The skin feels warm and firm (evidence of swelling under the skin.)

Prognosis

Reversible if you remove the pressure right away.

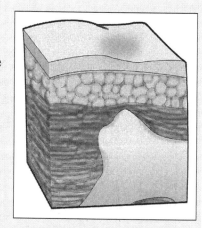

STAGE II
Description and Symptoms

A blister or a superficial loss of skin appearing as an abrasion or shallow crater. It may be painful and visibly swollen.

Prognosis

If the pressure is removed, the ulcer can heal in a relatively short time.

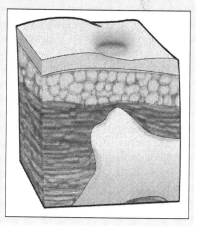

STAGE III
Description and Symptoms
A deep crater develops in the skin. Foul-smelling yellow or green fluid may ooze from it if there is infection present. The center is usually not painful because the nerve cells are dead.

Prognosis
It may take months to heal.

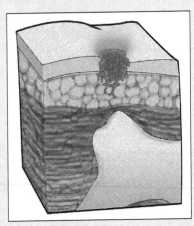

STAGE IV
Description and Symptoms
Tissue is now destroyed from the skin to the bone or close to the bone.

Prognosis
It usually takes a lot of time and costly treatment to heal.

It is important that you understand the various stages of pressure ulcer development. Inspecting the skin for early signs of an ulcer is critical for prevention.

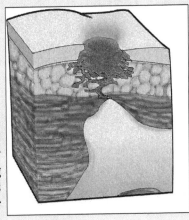

If a pressure ulcer is beginning to develop, your speedy response to the warning signs can prevent the development of a much more difficult wound.

When the early signs of a pressure ulcer are detected – even though you have carried out the instructions you were given – there may be a worsening of the condition before it gets better.

To ensure early detection and treatment, report any of the following to your nurse or physician:

- ☐ Reddened skin areas
- ☐ Blisters on the skin
- ☐ Rashes or skin inflammation
- ☐ Dry or rough skin
- ☐ Drainage or pus
- ☐ Bruises on the skin
- ☐ Pain or soreness
- ☐ Breaks or sores on the skin
- ☐ Scabs
- ☐ Swelling anywhere on the skin
- ☐ Loss of appetite
- ☐ White areas of the skin that are sore to the touch

IF YOU ARE A CAREGIVER

This book focuses on the needs of people who, for one reason or another, may be prone to skin problems. You may be cooperating with a medical team in the treatment of skin conditions such as pressure ulcers and you may have become quite knowledgeable concerning the many practical aspects of treatment. On the other hand, you may be in the situation where you have a loved one who's been assessed as being at risk of developing such problems and you simply want to help prevent this from happening.

Notes

In any caregiving procedure, the focus is naturally on the patient, perhaps to the emotional detriment of the caregiver. You have to ensure that you do not become a victim of the situation. As a caregiver, you can be consumed by ever-increasing demands on your time and capacity, and over a long period of time the process can be extremely stressful and emotionally draining. Because of this, we suggest you try to abide by the following general principles:

Encourage independence on the part of your patient.
It is important that your patient uses as much of his or her capabilities as possible. You need to strike a delicate balance of providing help when needed without inhibiting the self-reliance so vital for a person's morale, dignity and overall physical and mental health.

Take care of yourself.
You will be less effective as a caregiver if you neglect yourself. You must be especially aware of negative stress and take time to relax and do the things you enjoy. Inevitably, there will be conflict. It can be difficult to maintain a calm demeanor at all times and nobody expects you to do so. Instead of repressing your feelings when things get difficult, try to share them with others.

Don't be afraid to ask for help.
There are organizations, products, trained specialists and other resources available to help share the burden. Keep an open mind when seeking help, and don't feel like a "failure" for doing so. We have included a list of resources and websites at the end of this book.

Section 2
Treatment By Prevention

INTRODUCTION

Prevention of pressure ulcers is the number one treatment. Whatever dressings, medication, surgery or creams the nurse or doctor may use in treating a pressure ulcer, they will all be wasted unless preventive habits for the patient are developed and practiced!

This is not to diminish the importance of medical treatment. It is vital, especially for the advanced pressure ulcer. However, unlike most medical conditions, the patient can really help herself by co-operating with a careful, appropriately planned, preventive program that is thoroughly implemented.

The preventive program should be devised by you and your health care team. The needs of each patient will vary considerably. The most obvious variable is the degree of activity or mobility a patient has – a person with little control over his movements will need more involvement from the caregiver than a person will who is still relatively mobile.

In the following sections we'll attempt to inform you on how to prevent pressure ulcers developing or getting worse. The guidelines are not dangerous or controversial but we emphasize that each person's list of preventive measures should be worked out with a health care practitioner.

Notes

The more the patient can be involved in his or her treatment, the better. Besides reducing the caregiver's workload, patient involvement is an important psychological benefit: it enhances feelings of dignity, self-reliance and hope. Therefore, when it's appropriate, patient education should be an integral part of the preventive program.

Remember the old saying – "an ounce of prevention is worth a pound of cure!"

PRESSURE RELIEF

Unequalized pressure causes pressure ulcers. Put simply, if you can redistribute the excessive pressure on high-risk body areas, pressure ulcers will not develop; if they are already present, redistributing that pressure may help to bring about healing.

The objective of pressure redistribution is to maintain adequate blood flow at high-risk pressure points. This can be achieved in two ways: a) patient movement and repositioning, and b) use of pressure redistribution devices.

PATIENT MOVEMENT AND REPOSITIONING
- If possible, get the patient out of bed as often as you can.
- Exercise the patient's joints and muscles regularly to relieve pressure and stimulate circulation.
- Change the position of a wheelchair, chairbound or bedbound patient every half-hour, making sure to reposition the coccyx (tailbone) and hip pressure points.
- Encourage the patient to move around independently and change position as often as possible.
- When in bed, the patient's head should be only slightly elevated to spread the body weight over a wider surface and prevent sliding downward in the bed (causing shearing).
- Completely turn the patient (at least every two hours). This relieves skin pressure and irritation, promotes comfort and

stimulates blood circulation. Turning should alternate between resting on the back, on the side, on the stomach and then again on the back. This schedule should be linked to the positions that are the most comfortable for carrying out various necessary activities during the day. (For example, the patient should be lying on his or her back for meals.)

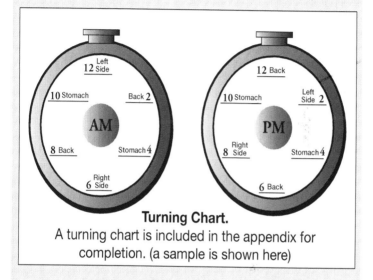

Turning Chart.
A turning chart is included in the appendix for completion. (a sample is shown here)

THE DO'S AND DON'TS OF TURNING AND REPOSITIONING

•**DO** encourage patient independence whenever possible. The effort can help improve overall health.

•**DO** keep a supply of pillows, towels and protective devices handy. Use these items appropriately to protect high-risk areas.

•**DO** make sure the patient is comfortable after turning or repositioning.

•**DON'T** accidentally knock or bump an existing sore or high-risk area during movement.

•**DON'T** leave a patient in an upright sitting position for long periods. This can create shearing forces.

•**DON'T** let a patient's feet rest directly against an unpadded footboard.

- **DON'T** leave a bedpan in position for a long time. The pressure could cause a sore within minutes.
- **DON'T** overstrain yourself. Get help if necessary.

POSITIONING A PATIENT IN BED

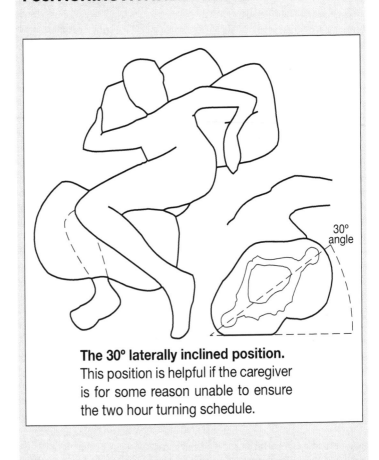

30°
angle

The 30° laterally inclined position.
This position is helpful if the caregiver
is for some reason unable to ensure
the two hour turning schedule.

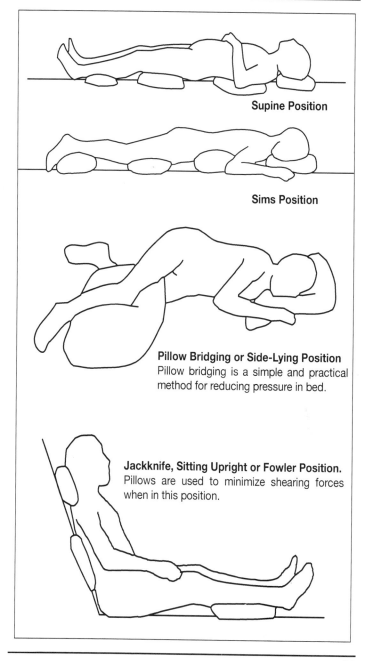

Supine Position

Sims Position

Pillow Bridging or Side-Lying Position
Pillow bridging is a simple and practical
method for reducing pressure in bed.

Jackknife, Sitting Upright or Fowler Position.
Pillows are used to minimize shearing forces
when in this position.

POSITIONING A PATIENT IN A WHEELCHAIR

A wheelchair is much more confining and limiting than a bed. The body weight must be shifted at least every 1 to 1½ hours.

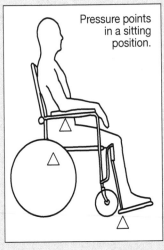

Pressure points in a sitting position.

If necessary, help reposition the patient's body so that his or her weight is shifted first to one buttock and then to the other. The changed position should be held for at least one minute.

If the patient can use her arms, encourage her to do push-ups in her chair. This can be done by gripping the chair arms and pressing down hard with her hands to raise her body off the seat. The use of pressure-distributing chair pads can be very beneficial.

Movement can be painful for the patient. When changing a patient's position or encouraging him to reposition himself, there may be some discomfort and consequent reluctance to move. Try to create some sort of mental distraction to keep his mind off the pain. Encourage him to think of a happy experience in his life or to imagine a pleasant, enjoyable setting. By putting aside the present and thinking pleasant thoughts, the discomfort and pain factor can be greatly minimized.

PRESSURE RELIEF PRODUCTS

Notes

Your health care practitioner may have recommended a pressure redistribution device in order to minimize the pressure and stress on your skin. There are many products on the market and only your health care professional can determine which is the correct one for you to use. As we have emphasized, the needs of each patient are unique and there are many factors that determine which device or product suits a particular patient.

The intent of the following section is to review what is available with regard to each type of product.

Also, it must be emphasized that your local home care dealer usually has a comprehensive selection of products and can always get you a particular product from the manufacturer.

Whether a pressure ulcer has already begun to develop or you are at risk of developing one, redistributing the pressure is the single most important factor.

FACTORS THAT CONTRIBUTE TO UNEQUALIZED PRESSURE ON THE BODY

- Weight of the body
- Frame of the body (square inches of the body surface)
- Characteristics of the support surface (flexibility, softness, ability to conform to body contours, density and hardness)
- Depth of device, be it a mattress or whatever

EXAMPLES OF COMMONLY USED DEVICES

Each patient has unique needs or issues, such as comfort, skin health, lifestyle and abilities, overall health and patient/caregiver acceptability of the proposed devices. Careful assessment of the individual risk factors together with the specific benefits of these devices needs to be integrated into the choice of device.

As a preventive measure, the Braden Scale for Predicting Pressure Sore Risk® is a clinically validated tool that allows nurses and other health care providers to predicts patients who are at risk for developing ulcers. (See www.bradenscale.com.)

Devices can be categorized as "low tech" and "high tech", here are some examples:

Low tech mattresses

- Standard foam mattresses – These are the least expensive choice. Density and hardness are critical factors, too little density can make the surface 'bottom out" or too much hardness can create peaks, creating localized high pressure on the skin. Further care should be taken to ensure trapped body heat does not cause excessive perspiration and any open sores should not touch the foam.

- Gel – filled mattresses – adjusts to the contours of the body.

- Air – filled mattresses / overlays

- Water – filled mattresses – these have an excellent ability to adjust to the contours of the body

- Tempur – Pedic® mattresses – this new material developed from the NASA program has proven pressure relieving qualities.

High tech mattresses

•Alternating pressure mattress / overlays – they work by increasing the surface area in contact with the skin.

•Turning beds/ frames –these motorized units reposition the patient

•Therapeutic Support systems – The AtmosAir® family of products offer KCI's proprietary Self Adjusting Technology™ (SAT™). <u>SAT™ is an "open-pressurize"</u> system that delivers non-powered, dynamic pressure-redistribution automatically and rapidly distributing body weight minimizing tissue interface pressure. The clinically proven AtmosAir® product line can help you achieve your clinical goals (lower incidence rate of pressure ulcers; treatment of individual pressure ulcers) and financial objectives.

As a footnote to the efficacy of these devices, it is interesting to note that the incidence and prevalence of heel ulcers appear to be increasing, especially among patients with diabetes, poor or limited mobility, peripheral vascular disease or who are otherwise at risk. A study was conducted comparing immobilized hip fracture patients who were receiving high-level nursing care and using an absolute pressure-relieving device – the HEELIFT® suspension boot – with patients who received the same level of care but did not use the boot. The study recorded zero heel ulcers among patients using the HEELIFT® suspension boot whereas 17% of the other group (receiving just nursing care) acquired heel ulcers. If pillows are being used to redistribute heel pressure, be careful the foot does not drop and cause damage, especially if a foot prop is not being used.

Appropriate Pressure
Relief Devices

Notes

_____

_____

_____

_____

_____

_____

_____

_____

_____

_____

_____

_____

_____

_____

_____

_____

_____

_____

SKIN CARE

The objective of skin care is to maintain and improve skin health to avoid pressure ulcers developing.

Important skin care tips

Inspection: Anybody at risk should have a systematic skin inspection at least once a day, paying particular attention to bony prominences. Observations should always be documented. (see skin care record in appendix). A simple peel –and-stick label that can be adhered to a patient's chart has been developed by Sage Products. This label has an outline of the human body and you can circle areas of concern.

Skin cleansing: This should occur at the time of soiling and at routine intervals. The frequency of skin cleansing should be individualized according to patient needs and preference.
Avoid hot water, and use only mild cleansing - agents that minimize irritation and dryness of the skin. Consider the use of a recommended skin cleanser. Towel - dry gently to avoid damaging the skin. If a person is overweight, dry the skin inside folds by directing the cool setting of a hand – held dryer over the area while you hold the skin folds apart.

Avoid dry skin: This can make the skin more vulnerable to damage. The two environmental causes to avoid can be low humidity (less than 40%) and exposure to cold. The use of a topical moisturizer can help alleviate dry skin.

Avoid massage over bony prominences: There is evidence to suggest that any improvement in circulation is outweighed by the real risk of skin damage.

Minimize exposure to moisture: Incontinence, perspiration or wound drainage can put the skin at risk for chafing, irritation, cracking or infection of the skin and it is vital to minimize this problem. It is well proven that the use of modern underpads that absorb moisture and present a quick drying surface with the skin can help and are preferable to products made of cloth. A further intervention that can help protect the skin is the use of professionally recommended moisture protectant creams or ointments.

Skin injury: This can be caused by physical shear or friction forces and can be minimized through proper positioning, transferring and turning techniques. In addition, friction injuries can be reduced by the use of lubricants, protective films / dressings and protective padding. Common sense tips like keeping sheets and other bed linen wrinkle - free and avoid spilling crumbs onto the bed. Also keep nails short to discourage scratching and discourage walking barefoot.

Skin Care Checklist:

Inspect & document skin daily ☐

Underpads, briefs or other
disposable incontinence care products ☐

Moisturizer product ☐

Moisture protectant product ☐

Skin cleanser product ☐

Optimum room temperature & humidity ☐

Avoidance measures for skin injury ☐

HYGIENE

Encourage a person to perform as much of his or her own hygiene practices as is possible. As well as keeping one clean, this can:
- Help fight infection.
- Maintain normal body temperature.
- Make the person more comfortable and relaxed.
- Boost morale (when you look your best you feel better emotionally and physically).
- Enhance healthy skin.
- Prevent skin irritation.

PERSONAL HYGIENE

Ensure recommended baths or showers are taken. If you are unsure of the general guidelines for giving baths, check with your nurse or physician.

If there is a problem concerning incontinence (leakage of urine or bowel waste from time to time), a physician or nurse will generally take specific measures to ease the problem. After incontinence it is important to get the skin clean and dry again. Use a mild, unscented soap, a specially formulated perineal cleaner or a heavy based ointment as recommended by your health professional to gently and effectively remove urine and stool.

After diarrhea, cleanse the anal region. There are preparations available that can be applied around the anus to prevent and treat the irritation.

The use of underpads that can absorb moisture and present a quick drying interface with the skin can dramatically solve the problem of incontinence and subsequent poor hygiene.

UNDERGARMENTS

These should be changed every day and immediately after exercise. It is important to ensure that they are the right size; preferably, they should be made of cotton, and light and soft in texture. Your home care dealer or nurse will recommend the optimum quality products.

Notes

If elastic stockings or bandages are used, the same hygiene policies should be implemented. With these, however, it is very important that they fit properly to avoid irritation and restricted blood flow.

BED LINEN
The choice of bed linen is important – the patient should not be too warm or be allowed to perspire. Sheets and pillowcases should be clean, dry and soft and free of creases to ensure comfort. Always wipe food crumbs from bed linen after each meal.

In a case where the bedwear is irritating sensitive pressure points, applying a preventive dressing can minimize the danger.

In concluding this section on skin care, it is important to appreciate that all aspects of caring for the skin must be addressed; one weak link in the chain can ruin all of your good efforts.

NUTRITION AND HYDRATION

Proper nutrition is an important factor in preventing and treating ulcers. Ensuring patients receive adequate nutrients and water/fluid reduces the risk of developing pressure ulcers as well as contributing significantly to the healing process. The blood in our bodies carries vital oxygen and nutrients to the cells; to make sure there is enough blood, you have to drink enough fluids. Usually drinking 8 glasses of water every day will achieve this, unless the patient is on a fluid restricted diet.

The body needs extra energy (calories), tissue-building components (protein) and other nutrients to heal damaged tissue and resist infection. To achieve this, a professional dietitian can provide a high calorie diet, rich in proteins and other important nutrients. It's helpful to have appetizing meals and use appropriate plates and utensils. Check the health of the mouth, especially the teeth, to ensure there are no vitamin deficiencies.

As malnutrition is a major risk factor, early screening and assessment are critical. If a patient has lost more than 10% of his normal body weight in the past 6 months or 5% of his weight within the past month, he may be at risk of malnutrition. Another important benchmark to evaluate the nutritional health of a patient is to measure the amount of albumin in the body . Albumin is a protein manufactured by the liver and it performs many vital functions such as ensuring optimum transportation of nutrients to the cells. There are other reasons for a low albumin level, but a level of less than 3.0 mg/dL is considered a risk factor for poor nutritional status. Malnutrition and poor hydration are the most common reasons for the pressure ulcer condition.

The dietitian will consider the following key needs for a balanced diet, to maintain weight or promote weight gain:

Adequate calories
(30 - 40 calories per kilogram of body weight);

High protein levels
(1.2 – 2.0 g per kilogram of body weight)

Adequate levels of vitamins A, C and E, and zinc will ensure immune function, collagen formation and protein metabolism.

Arginine is an amino acid, found in dairy, meat, poultry and fish. Its role in wound healing encompasses cells dividing properly, facilitating immune function, promoting the secretion of key hormones, promoting collagen synthesis and indirectly keeping blood vessels dilated to help in oxygen transfer. Its importance often necessitates using a supplemental source.

Dietary nucleotides and omega-3 fatty acids (found in fish like sardines, mackerel, salmon) also contribute to a healthy immune system.

Adequate water/fluid intake is needed to maintain fluid status and transport oxygen, nutrients and growth factors to the site of the pressure ulcer.

Many patients at risk for pressure ulcers are known to have poor diets. Consequently the use of supplements can be of enormous benefit if a deficiency is suspected or established. The dietitian or health care practitioner can recommend appropriate supplements and other actions. See the nutrition guidelines in the Appendix.

COMFORT MEASURES

From time to time, in the midst of all the attention paid to the treatment regimen of dressing changes, pressure-relieving rituals and skin care, the comfort of the patient can be overlooked.

When the patient is comfortable, he feels at ease with himself and his surroundings. He'll be more willing to comply with treatment and more receptive to suggestions on how to help with prevention efforts. Every effort should be made – especially with a less mobile patient or someone in pain – to increase the patient's comfort level.

During an acute phase of a pressure ulcer condition, a person feels more comfortable if she gets the right amount of the following essentials:

A. Uninterrupted sleep
B. Rest and relaxation
C. Movement, exercise and activity
D. Relief from pain

A. UNINTERRUPTED SLEEP

Without proper sleep, even healthy people tend to not have the energy to participate in some daily activities. In the extreme, for an at risk patient, this can effect well-being, which in turn can affect a person's desire to take care of himself. A person who is not sleeping well may also not eat well or drink enough fluids, factors that have a direct link to the development of pressure ulcers and impaired wound healing. There is also clinical evidence that lack of sleep is a serious contributor to dementia.

We all know how refreshing a good night's rest can be. This is because during sleep certain hormones enter the blood stream and help keep the nervous system in good working order, help fight infection and help heal and repair body tissues. So as well as helping the healing process of the skin, sleep helps the patient feel less irritable, more alert and generally more positive about recovery. Individual requirements vary greatly but most people operate best on seven or eight hours a night. What's normal for one person may be too much or too little for another, so if you naturally wake up after five or six hours and can't fall back to sleep, don't worry – you probably don't need more sleep. Keep in mind also that as we age our sleep patterns change.

The important aspect of sleep is quality of sleep. Normally, sleep occurs in 90-minute cycles. During a typical cycle, periods of shallow and deep sleep alternate with rapid eye movement (REM) sleep, during which time dreams occur. It's not known what role dreams play, but we do know that we need our REM sleep for emotional well being.

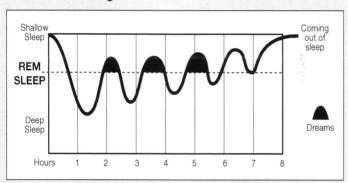

So just when you need as much sleep as possible to help heal pressure ulcers, you may find that because of pain, turning schedules and so on, your sleep patterns are always being disturbed. The following tips may be helpful but always check with your medical team if in doubt.

Choosing the right mattress

This should be a priority; in fact, your health care practitioner may have recommended one of the product types listed in the "pressure redistribution" section of this book. Often your mattress may have exceeded its life expectancy – about 9-10 years for most quality mattresses. Again it must be emphasized "pressure redistribution" is the objective. More specifically, any fluid type support surface that conforms easily to the contours of the body is best. The popular Tempur-Pedic® brand developed from the NASA program deserves a special mention as fulfilling the critical criteria.

How to sleep better

- If you nap during the day, try to nap in the morning, not the afternoon. A morning nap usually consists of REM sleep and generally leaves you feeling more refreshed. Also, if you nap in the morning you will be more likely to feel tired enough by the evening to fall asleep.
- If your condition permits, try to get some exercise during the day so that you will feel tired by bedtime.
- If your doctor has prescribed pain medication, you may check to see if it's okay to take it during the night so the pain doesn't wake you up.
- Get into the ritual of performing the same activities in the same order each night before you go to bed. This will tell your body it's time for sleep.
- Help your body relax by taking a warm bath or shower each night before you go to bed. If this is not possible, ask a family member or a friend to give you a soothing back rub.
- Make sure you are neither too hot nor too cold before bedtime.
- If restlessness keeps you awake during the night, watch TV or get out of bed if possible and do something until you start to feel drowsy. Then return to bed and try to sleep.
- Finish eating 2-3 hours before bedtime.
- Avoid nicotine (cigarettes, tobacco products), caffeine (coffee, tea, soft drinks, chocolate) and alcohol, at least 3 hours before bedtime.
- Make your bedroom sleep-conducive – cool, quiet, dark and comfortable. Remove the TV, computers and general clutter.

B. REST AND RELAXATION

This is a very individual matter. Some people prefer their surroundings to be quiet and private; others may like a certain type of music as background sound. There are plenty of books and self-help manuals that can help you not only find the right approach but train yourself to achieve a relaxed state. Some well-proven approaches include:

Focusing your thoughts

Choose a word, sound or phrase and repeat it silently or aloud. If distracting thoughts arise, try to disregard them and continue concentrating.

Notes

Progressive muscle relaxation

This involves tensing and relaxing individual muscle groups. Begin by making sure you find a time when you won't be disturbed. Now close your eyes. Focus on a muscle group such as your hand muscles. Tense your forearm muscles and make a fist. Notice how the sensation feels. After six to eight seconds, release your fist and relax your muscles. Concentrate on the different feeling you experience when your muscles relax.

Now concentrate on a different muscle group. Continue until you've tensed and relaxed all your muscle groups in turn. Take a systematic approach. When you've completed the exercise, open your eyes. You will feel as if you're awakening from a deep sleep.

Guided imagery

There are commercial recordings that teach guided imagery techniques. The process is like daydreaming except that you make a more deliberate, controlled effort. The general guidelines include:

- Find a comfortable position, draw the blinds and dim the lights – get rid of all distractions.
- Decide how long you want the session to last (usually 15 – 20 minutes).
- Choose a pleasant, relaxing image – a beach scene, perhaps, one that you've actually experienced and can recall fairly easily.
- Try to relax by taking long, deep breaths.
- Focus on imagining every detail of the scene, i.e. seagulls, the waves rolling in, the sand under your feet, the warmth of the sun on your body. Above all, imagine how relaxed and peaceful you feel in these surroundings.
- After 15 minutes or so you should be in a state of relaxation.

Notes

There are many other ways to help you relax – massage and hypnosis, for example. Ask your nurse or caregiver to help you find the technique most suited to you and your particular situation.

C. MOVEMENT AND EXERCISE

You must appreciate that everybody is unique in the activities they can carry out to help in recovery. Your medical team can advise you on this. The degree of mobility you have is a key factor in determining your activities and exercise level. If you are spending most of your time in bed, a basic objective will be to prevent stiff joints and muscle weakness. The following are tips for improving your level of physical activity:

To prevent stiff joints

Try to move each joint through its entire range of motion every hour or so when you are awake. Wiggle your toes and flex your fingers. Rotate your wrists and ankles. Check with your physician or nurse as to how often and to what extent you should do this.

Gently squeeze a foam rubber ball or rolled-up washcloth to prevent hand stiffness.

If you feel pain or resistance at any time when you move your joints, stop right away. Tell your caregiver or physician where and when your joints hurt.

To prevent muscle weakness

Practice tightening and relaxing your muscles to help keep them strong. Don't hold your breath as you tighten your muscles – just breathe normally.

Ask your medical team about isometric exercises you can perform in bed that might be useful to you.

If your doctor says it's okay, try to get out of bed as soon as you can. Don't stay in bed longer than you have to. This gets the blood circulating and your body "perks up."

When carrying out these activities make sure you do not cause any trauma (such as a knock or a scrape) to your pressure ulcer. This could considerably set back your healing process so it is a primary consideration in your exercise plan. There are special dressings that serve as protective covering against pressure ulcer trauma.

Notes

D. RELIEF FROM PAIN

It is the caregiver or patient's right to demand attention to this comfort issue because it can affect sleep, mobility, compliance to treatment and sometimes bring on depression. This is a major quality of life issue for the patient and can affect healing times. Many marginalized patients, like the elderly and the immobile, live with the pain without complaining. A recent study showed that even though 62% of patients were suffering chronic leg ulcer pain, nurses assessed the pain in only 7% of the patients.

Pain from a wound can have different causes requiring different types of medications prescribed by your doctor. Some tips when taking oral medication include:

Be sure to follow the dosage regimen and your doctor's advice always to the letter.
Don't wait until you are in a lot of pain before taking your medication. Be proactive.
Check with your doctor if the following occurs: a) your pain is bad in the morning, b) your medication makes you feel sleepier than usual, c) your pain seems different, or d) you become constipated.
Make sure you check with your doctor or nurse as to what may negatively interact with your medication, such as alcohol, other drugs, herbs etc.

In 2006, Canada saw the launch of the first dressing with built-in pain relief medication, which is delivered directly to the wound surface. Biatain – Ibu is not only capable of absorbing wound exudates but continuously releases ibuprofen, the drug in brands such as Motrin and Advil, to the wound site only, without circulating in the body and possibly causing side effects.

Notes

For more information visit www.coloplast.ca or www.biatain-ibu. coloplast.com. Here you will find practical information for wound patients and their families. Plus, there is a section for health care professionals which provides many helpful guides to wound care and practical pain assessment downloads.

CONCLUSION

For the caregiver, making sure your patient is comfortable could be the catalyst to bring about better patient cooperation and an improved quality of life. Make sure you have an open dialogue and listen carefully to her concerns.

COMFORT CHECK LIST:

GETTING ENOUGH SLEEP:
Get a new mattress ☐
Read self help tips to better sleep habits. ☐

REST AND RELAXATION:
Warmth ☐   Background music ☐
Breathing exercises ☐   Hypnosis ☐
Guided Imagery ☐   Muscle Relaxation ☐
TENS (Electrical stimulation) ☐ Biofeedback ☐

MOVEMENT AND EXERCISE
Isometric exercises ☐
R.O.M. (Range Of Motion) exercises ☐
Plan not to "knock" your ulcer ☐

RELIEF FROM PAIN
Know your prescribed medication ☐
Read self help medication tips ☐
Tell your Dr. or caregiver about pain ☐
Ask for pain relief medication ☐
Ask about Biatain –Ibu pain relief dressing ☐
Visit www.biatain-ibu.coloplast.com ☐

GENERAL PREVENTIVE TIPS

Notes

•Prevent accidents and falls by organizing the home sensibly and ensuring that routinely used equipment is well maintained.

•Smoking in bed at night should be forbidden and patients who do smoke should wear a protective apron.

•Keep essentials such as a bedpan, light switch, bell and so on near the bed and within reach.

•Ensure all personal appliances, crutches, walkers and wheelchairs are properly fitted, comfortable and well maintained.

•Rubber-soled footwear should always be used.

•An appropriate footstool should be available near the bed.

•Floors should be kept dry and clean.

•Do all you can to ensure a feeling of comfort, security and safety in order for the patient to maintain emotional well being.

TAKING CARE IN THE HOME

If you are caring for someone who is suffering from muscle weakness, loss of coordination or balance problems, you should make some changes to your living space. A normal home can be unexpectedly hazardous – a minor slip or fall can worsen an existing skin ulcer.

Ask your nurse, occupational therapist, physician or appropriate health care professional for advice on your home's safety and convenience. Here are some general points for home safety:

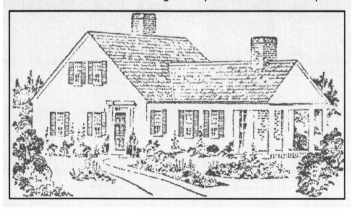

The Bathroom

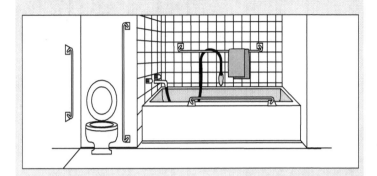

☐ Grab bars and a tub seat are helpful for getting in or out of the bath.

☐ A shower chair can allow the patient to sit in the shower.

☐ An elevated toilet for easier usage.

☐ Non-slip mats in the bathtub or shower.

☐ A hand-held shower will make washing and rinsing much easier.

☐ A night light can prevent knocks.

☐ Lower mirrors and shelves if the person is in a wheelchair.

The Bedroom

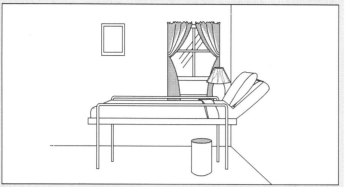

❏ A hospital bed with side rails and attached trapeze can be helpful. Make sure casters or wheels are locked or removed.

❏ If necessary raise the bed about 4 inches to make it the same height as a wheelchair.

❏ Position the bed against a wall to help make it stationary.

❏ Have a telephone near the bed and a bell to call for help.

❏ Provide a night light, and keep a flashlight near the bed in case of emergency.

❏ Organize the room so the patient can have an outside view.

❏ Replace thick or shag carpets with low-pile carpet to make movement easier.

The Kitchen

❏ Remove rugs to prevent slips.

❏ Avoid excessive waxing of floors.

❏ Reorganize storage for easier access.

❏ Make sure the stove has controls that are easy to reach.

Notes

Section 3
Pressure Ulcer Treatment

A healing pressure ulcer – or any wound – is an extremely complex and dynamic tissue for which scientific researchers and clinicians are continually acquiring new knowledge and different effective treatments.

Healing occurs in recognizable phases, which are usually progressive, and often overlapping. This is a collaborative process involving a wide variety of cells and components which need to continually interact in order for the skin to heal. This is the realm of cellular and molecular research and is not really appropriate for the more generalist nature of this book.

In more general terms there are certain factors that influence healing and it's worth pinpointing these so that the various treatment options make sense to you.

FACTORS THAT INFLUENCE HEALING

Moisture/Humidity

Maintaining a moist wound environment has been proven to assist the healing process, providing the following advantages: a) prevents tissue dehydration, helping to stop the formation of a scab or dry crust (eschar) on the top of the wound. This eschar can hinder the migration of newly-formed skin cells (the technical name is epithelial cells) to the surface of the skin. These new cells can only move through the thin watery liquid within the wound – that liquid is called the serous exudate; b) increases the growth of new blood vessels; c) assists in the interaction of the growth factors in the target cells; d) reduces the chances of infection, and e) is associated with less pain.

Notes

Debridement
This is the technical term for removing any blood clots, scabs or dry crust on the wound. This can be achieved by the following four methods: a) surgical – removing tissue using a scalpel or scissors; b) mechanical – referring to a range of techniques like wet-to-dry dressings, wound irrigation or whirlpool or foot soaks; c) enymatic – using collagens, and d) autolytic – using certain dressings like hydrogels which enhance the body's own enzymes. Debridement is needed to ensure a moist wound environment in order for the wound to heal.

Tissue exudate
Secretions of fluid are produced by the inflammatory response of the wound/pressure ulcer. This exudate actively promotes healing through its nutrients and provides an ideal fluid for the new skin cells to move or migrate to the new skin "building sites."

Temperature
Wounds should be kept covered to maintain optimum physiological temperatures. Cleansing agents should be used at body temperature.

Infection
As you would expect, infection slows down the healing process and extends the inflammatory response. Infections must be eliminated as soon as possible; the physician will use creams, ointments or antibiotics to clear up this problem.

Intrinsic factors
Advancing age, combined with a slower metabolic process and associated reduced collagen and poor circulation can impede the

healing process.

A range of disease processes can adversely affect the ability of the wound to heal; these include anemia, arteriosclerosis, cancer, cardiovascular disorders, diabetes, immune disorders, inflammatory diseases, liver problems, rheumatoid arthritis and uremia.

Psychological factors like stress and anxiety can also affect the immune system and can disturb sleep which is important for the healing of wounds.

Extrinsic factors

Malnutrition, smoking, certain drug therapies, radiotherapy and fluid balance can also affect the healing process.

The main point in the healing process is to remove all adverse influences. Nature has set a healing time for each type of wound and that healing will only occur if there is a favorable environment.

TREATMENT OPTIONS

DRESSINGS

Having reviewed the influential factors when it comes to wound or pressure sore healing, we will now review the available treatments. Each wound or pressure ulcer is unique, as is each patient; the health care practitioner, therefore, has to choose the products and treatment options that fit the situation.

The choice of dressing can not only influence the wound site environment but is also a preventive factor for both infection and trauma.

It's remarkable how health care companies have developed such a wide range of dressings for every stage of pressure ulcer. Some companies have a dressing for each stage and profile of pressure ulcer. Others have developed innovative features that help in difficult characteristics of the wound. One company produces a unique, natural dressing from saline; others have high tech dressings developed from synthetic compounds.

Notes

You can benefit from these innovations, but the choice of dressing is the domain of the physicians and nurses who are extremely skilled and experienced in choosing what is right for the patient.

By definition, a dressing is a clean or sterile covering applied directly to a wound. The characteristics of an ideal wound dressing are as follows: a) to maintain optimum moisture/humidity at the wound/dressing interface; b) to remove excess exudates; c) to allow gaseous exchange; d) to provide thermal insulation; e) to be impermeable to bacteria; f) to be free of particles and toxic wound contaminants, and g) to allow removal without causing trauma to the wound.

Before we attempt to explain the treatment principles linked to the various wound phases, we must appreciate certain psychological and practical factors in the choice of dressing.

Patient comfort helps motivate and boost the feeling of wellness. A patient is going to be more optimistic and willing to get involved in treatment when she is feeling comfortable, and a caregiver or nurse is more likely to achieve cooperation and compliance from a patient who is feeling physically comfortable. So the "comfort factor" needs to be taken into account when choosing a dressing.

We must also consider the nursing time involved and cost of the dressing. Clearly there are practical considerations, such as the availability of the nurse or caregiver and how the dressings are to be paid for, that must be considered as well.

A dressing's purpose can be to absorb secretions, protect the wound from trauma, cover the wound with a drug, keep the wound clean or stop bleeding. The range of dressings include absorbent dressings, antiseptic dressings, occlusive dressings, pressure dressings and wet dressings. It's important to appreciate the critical importance of dressings because of their intimate contact with the wound.

There is no universally appropriate dressing – each is designed for a particular stage of healing and it is difficult to provide a simple formula in a booklet like this. Again, we emphasize that the physician and nurse are the only people who can decide what is appropriate for each unique wound.

However, you may find it helpful to review the modern approach in attempting to classify wounds with regard to the "right" sort of dressing. In Section I, under How to Recognize a Pressure Ulcer, we described the four stages – or phases – of pressure ulcers. Certain dressings are appropriate to these stages but for practical reasons we'd like to introduce you to another way of looking at pressure ulcers – categorizing them by the colors red, yellow and black.

The point of this book is to help you prevent pressure ulcers and help the healing process by the use of common sense techniques of prevention and management. We have emphasized the absolute decision-making role of the medical team in determining the proper course of treatment. Consequently, the following suggestions focus on principles of treatment, rather than products.

Pre-ulcerative lesion (reddened skin) phase

(This is a Stage I only category) In this phase there is usually no break in the skin; however, there are ominous signs of reddening and sometimes swelling and being warm to the touch. Unless appropriate basic intervention steps are taken, imminent tissue breakdown is a possibility.

This is perhaps the most definitive phase of pressure ulcers. It is the phase that is the most easily reversible through sensible intervention, perhaps by removing the source of pressure or friction/shearing and protecting the tissue from excessive moisture and further trauma. Improving the blood supply to the area could also help. Pivotal to the success of treatment is the basic care of the skin, using cleansers, moisturizers and/or protective creams and ointments.

Choice of dressing

The key issues are to protect the skin at all costs; to prevent further trauma, one should be able to remove the dressing without damaging the skin. The nature of the dressing should not encourage the "softening" (macerating) of both healthy and "at risk" skin but should support a healthy skin environment.

Granulation (red) phase

This dominant red appearance is evidence of a clean wound which is either ready to heal or is actually healing; the phase can actually overlap into Stages II, III and IV according to the severity of the pressure ulcer. The dominant theme of this phase is the obvious regenerative nature of the wound – new cell growth. It would be useful to review the classical appearance at each stage of this "granulation" phase:

Notes

Stage II – Only superficial tissue loss is apparent with skin loss occurring only in the epidermis or dermis (see Section I showing cross-section of the skin). The pressure ulcer could look like an abrasion, blister or shallow crater. This type of sore appears clean with a pink or red base or clusters of growing tissue. The drainage from the wound may be simply a thin, watery fluid (serous) or mixed with blood (serosanguinous).

Stage III – Damage now occurs to the subcutaneous tissue, showing itself as quite a deep crater. Again, because of the granulating or rapid healing process of skin growth, the wound appears clean with a pink to red bed or small granulating clusters. This time the serous or serosanguinous drainage may be not mild but heavy.

Stage IV – In this stage there is evidence of enormous tissue damage that can extend to muscle, bone or supporting structures such as the tendon or joint capsule. Again, there are both types of moderate to heavy fluid drainage.

Choice of dressing

In this active stage, dressings serve many purposes. Let's review the various factors:

•Maintaining a clean and moist environment. This is vital for cell growth and migration necessary for healing. The maintenance of a moist wound surface prevents wound desiccation (drying up) which is detrimental to the healing process.

•Absorbing excess exudate. Too much wound exudate can soften (macerate) surrounding tissues. In fact, large amounts of wound exudate can dilute wound healing factors and nutrients at the wound surface. Also, the toxins made by bacteria in the wound can further inhibit the wound repair process so the dressing should absorb these toxins to optimize the healing process.

•Protect newly-formed tissue. Obviously, any infection or trauma to the healing wound can delay recovery so it is very important that the dressing not stick to the wound surface and also protect the wound from the outside.

•Maintain a thermally-insulated wound environment. Keeping normal tissue temperature improves blood flow to the wound bed and helps in cell migration.

•Obliterate "dead space". By dead space, we mean the areas of empty space between the skin surface and wound floor, underlying intact surface tissues.

Clearly, there are dressings that fulfill these criteria and should be used as instructed by the manufacturer. Aggressive treatment at this phase can halt the progression to the inflammation and necrotic phases which are more difficult to treat. Site management usually involves cleaning the wound with saline solution.

Inflammatory (yellow) phase

This is a highly active phase with an obvious yellow fibrous debris or thick surface exudate present. Granulation tissue may be visible but the major concern here is looking for signs of infection. Wound drainage will be moderate to heavy and pus may be present.

Inflammation and infection are extremely problematical in delaying the healing process and the choice of dressing is critical when tackling these problems. Again, site management will call for cleansing the wound with saline but debris will also have to be removed, either mechanically or with assistance from an appropriate wound product.

Choice of dressing

Again, let's review the key factors:

Notes

•Supporting the natural cleansing mechanism of the wound. Keeping the wound clean is vital to ensure there is no further exacerbation of infection.

•Absorbing excess exudate. Too much exudate can soften (macerate) the surrounding skin and make it vulnerable. Dilution of wound healing factors and nutrients can slow down the healing process. It is important that in this phase, a dressing be able to absorb bacterial toxins.

•Supporting the removal of necrotic (dead) or foreign tissue from the wound. This can prevent further inflammation.

•Discouraging bacterial growth. This will help to reduce infection.

Necrotic (black) phase

The wound may now be partially or completely covered with black eschar (dry crust) or with loose or string-like necrotic tissue, which may be black, brown or gray in color. There may be purulent (pus-like) or fibrous material at the edges of the wound. Necrotic wounds can fall into stage II, III or IV categories.

This black phase is usually quite advanced and considerable site management is necessary. Besides the usual cleansing with saline, it is vital to remove the debris (debridement) of necrotic tissue. Dead tissue can cause further inflammation and/or provide an environment for bacterial growth, as well as slowing down the healing process. It is up to the medical team to decide how this tissue should be debrided from the wound.

Choice of dressing

There are many options for this category. Obviously, it is very important to choose a dressing that provides effective debridement as well as minimizing the risk of infection.

TYPES OF DRESSING

Your medical team will provide a dressing designed to meet the specific needs of your pressure ulcer/wound. There is no one dressing available that can provide a perfect environment for all wounds. Most clinicians, with this in mind, have an arsenal of dressings, so they can choose the right dressing for the right patient at the right time. Try to be an informed consumer with regard to dressings because the clinician will find your comments helpful when it comes to the following matters:

Any pain you may experience during dressing changes.

Any discomfort you may feel.

Whether you find any odors from the wound offensive or perhaps offensive to family members.

Always tell the clinician about any odors from the wound because it could mean a change of dressing is necessary to fight infection.

Do you consider yourself at risk from damaging the wound? If so, protection may be required.

Find out if you and your clinician agree on how many times the dressing should be changed and the length of time it will take to heal.

Here are the various categories of dressings with some common brand names included. This classification is not a rigid one as, in practice, there are many hybrid or composite dressings that combine aspects of members of different groups in order to achieve an optimum effect:

Transparent films

These are polyurethane based and transparent with varying thickness and adhesive coatings on one side only (to adhere to the skin). These dressings are impermeable to bacteria and fungi but can be permeated by moisture and oxygen. Brand names: Sure Site™, Tegaderm™, Carrafilm™, Comfeel®, Bioclusive*, Transeal®, Polyskin® and OpSite*.

Gauzes and non-woven dressings

These are available as sponges or wraps and, depending on their design, have varying degrees of absorbency. They are made of cotton, rayon or polyester and are available as sterile or non-sterile. Brand names: Curity Gauze Sponges, Carrington® Bordered Gauze, Avant Gauze™, CovRSite® Cover, Telfar, FLUFTEX™ and Medline® Bordered Gauze.

Soft silicone mesh

This is a non-adhering, porous, semi-transparent dressing with a wound contact layer consisting of flexible polyamide net coated with soft silicone. Although it is nonabsorbent, the porous nature allows fluid to pass through to the secondary dressing. Primarily used in skin donor sites. Brand name: Mepitel®.

Hydrocolloids

These are composed of carboxymethylcellulose (a sort of heavy carbohydrate), gelatin or pectin and have different absorption capabilities depending upon their thickness and composition. They are waterproof, impermeable to bacteria, promote autolytic debridement and can be changed every 3 to 7 days. Absorption, however, is limited. These are useful in granulating and epithializing wounds with minimal exudates. Brand names: Duo Derm®, Comfeel® Plus, 3M™ Tegasorb™, CaraColloid™, Procol®, Permacol™, Restore™, NU-DERM* BORDER, AquaTack™, ExuDERM™, CUTINOVA* Hydro, RepliCare® and Ultec®.

Alginates

These are non-woven sheets or ropes composed of natural polysaccharide fibers derived from seaweed. They are comfortable and good for heavy exuding wounds. However, they may cause drying of the wound if it is not producing enough fluid. Brand names: Kaltostat®, Curasorb®, Sorbsan®, 3M™ Tegagen™, SeaSorb® Soft, CarraGinate™, NU-DERM*, Maxorb™ Melgisorb®, AlgiSite*, and CURASORB®.

Biologicals and biosynthetics

These are gels, solutions or semi-occlusive sheets derived from a natural source. They act as sort of scaffolds to promote healing of the tissues. Brand names: Oasis®, BIOBRANE® and Apilagraf®.

Collagen dressings

These can be particles, sheets, and amorphous dressings; as the name implies, collagen is derived from animal sources. These dressings encourage the deposition and organization of newly formed collagen fibers and granulation tissue within the wound bed. Brand names: FIBRACOL* and PROMOGRAN*. and Woun'Dres®.

Cavity fillers

As the name suggests these dressings fill in dead space within the wound and can be in the form of beads, foam, gel, pillow, strand, ointment or paste. Their function is to keep the wound moist and absorb exudates. A secondary dressing for protection is required over the cavity filler. Brand names: Flexigel® Strands®, Carrasorb™ TRIAD™ and MULTIDEX®.

Absorptives

These are multilayered wound cover dressings that provide either a semi-adherent quality or non-adherent layer, combined with highly absorptive layers of fiber, such as cotton, rayon or cellulose. They are designed to minimize wound trauma and manage moderate exudates. Brand names: Mepore®, Covaderm®, Aquacel®, Primapore*, IODOFLEX™, SOFSORB®.

Contact layers

These are thin sheets of non-adherent material placed in the wound bed to protect granulating tissue from other potentially destructive dressings. These dressings conform to the shape of the wound bed and, being porous, allow wound fluids and exudates to flow through for absorption by a secondary dressing. Brand names: Mepitel®, 3M™ Tegapore™, Profore* and DERMANET®.

Foams

These are absorptive sheets and shapes of formed polymer solutions such as polyurethane, with small open cells, which hold fluids and have non-adherent layers. They are easy to apply and remove and are useful with wounds with large volumes of exudates. Some foam dressings are available in both non-adhesive and adhesive versions, the latter does not require a secondary dressing. Brand names: Allevyn*, Optifoam™, PolyMem®, 3M™ Foam Adhesive, Lyofoam®, POLYDERM™, Hydrofera Blue™, SOF-FOAM*, TIELLE*, Mepilex®, CURAFOAM® and Biatain™. Other foams are available that secure the dressing in place during application while minimizing trauma to granulation tissue on removal. Brand name: Biatain Soft-Hold.

Hydrogel dressings

These are primarily composed of water and are designed to donate moisture to the wound site. Some special formulas actually absorb exudates as well – a "smart" dressing. Brand names: Intrasite*, TenderWet®, SkinTegrity™ Hydrogel, 3M™ Tegagel™, Carrasmart™, Purilon™, DuoDERM®, Dermagran®, CURASOL®, NU- GEL*, IntraSite* and SoloSite®.

Impregnated dressings

These include gauzes and non-woven sponges, ropes and strips that are saturated with a solution, emulsion, oil agent or compound including saline, petroleum, zeroform, zinc salts, iodine or scarlet red. Brand names: Vaseline Petrolatum Gauze®, Adaptic* Non Adhering Dressing.

ACTIVE DRESSINGS
1)Silver dressings

These deliver a sustained release, broad spectrum, antimicrobial action while maintaining a moist environment for the wound. Available as many different dressing types, their objective is to treat or reduce the risk of infection. Brand names: Acticoat*, Arglaes®, SilvaSorb™ and Contreet®.

2) Pain relief

The only available brand, Biatain-Ibu, is a foam dressing with a built-in analgesic, Ibuprofen, which is delivered directly to the wound site, and thereby may relieve both temporary pain (during dressing change) and persistent pain, as well as manage the wound exudate.

Composites

These are wound covers that possess more than one component to address the multiple wound care needs and dressing functions. They can function as primary or secondary dressings. Brand names: Telfa® Plus Barrier Island, 3M™ Tegaderm™, Plus Pad Transparent dressing with absorbent pad, 3M™ Medipore™, COVADERMPLUS®, CovRSite® and TELFA®.

All these dressings try to address the major goals of providing cover, protection, hydration (keeping moist), insulation and absorption, as well as preventing infection, filling dead space, promoting granulation (healing) and debridement. Each category of dressing fits some or most of these needs; deciding which to use requires the skill and judgement of a health care practitioner.

The Agency for Health Care Policy and Research (AHCPR), which is the authoritative clinical body, has made critical dressing recommendations, the most important of which are as follows:

A dressing should keep the ulcer bed moist. Healing has been found to be faster when the wound bed is kept moist.

The skin surrounding the ulcer should be kept dry. This is to prevent the surrounding skin from becoming damaged.

A dressing, although absorbing exudates, should not dry out or desiccate the wound bed.

CHANGING A DRESSING

Pressure ulcers go through stages of healing. The physician or nurse will vary the selection, size and frequency of dressing change according to the type of wound. The following guidelines are for basic dressing change and cleaning procedures:

Put on gloves.

Remove all hand jewelry.

Wash your hands thoroughly before handling the gloves.

When you have both gloves on, check to be sure there are no breaks in the glove material. If you find any, discard the gloves and start again with a new set.

Applying a gauze dressing

If the person you're caring for has a draining bedsore, you'll need to change the dressing regularly. Begin by assembling your equipment: dressings (regular gauze or nonstick gauze pads), scissors, adhesive tape, cleaning solution prescribed by the doctor, baby oil and a plastic disposal bag. Have the new dressing ready before removing the old one. Cut strips of adhesive tape in advance. Before you start, position the person so you can easily reach the pressure ulcer.

Tip: If the doctor prescribes medication to make dressing changes less painful, give the medication to the patient 1/2 hour before changing the dressing.

Notes

Removing the old dressing

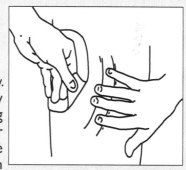

Wash your hands thoroughly. Remove the tape carefully from the patient's skin, leaving the old dressing in place for now. If necessary to make removal less painful, moisten the old tape with baby oil before you remove it. If the skin under the old tape is inflamed, don't apply the new tape there.

Remove the old dressing, but don't touch any part of it that touched the ulcer. Fold together the edges of the dressing, place it in the disposal bag and close the bag tightly.

Checking the ulcer

Check for swelling, redness, drainage, pus, all of which are signs of probable infection. Is the wound healing? Check the amount and color of drainage on the old dressing. Do not touch the ulcer. Whether the ulcer appears to be infected, healing or unchanged since the last dressing change, write down what you see; do this every time you change the dressing.

Important: Note the amount and color of any drainage.

Notes

FOR FURTHER INFORMATION ABOUT DRESSINGS

Manufacturers' Information

The manufacturers of these physician-approved and well-tested dressings have information on why they are used for a particular stage of a pressure ulcer as well as detailed instructions on how they are to be applied. Your pharmacist or home care store can provide the information you need and even refer you to the manufacturer.

Home Health Care Retail Stores

As a patient, caregiver or nurse these outlets can be a valuable resource in helping you prevent and treat skin problems.

There are usually highly competent staff to help you – often nurses who are aware of the principles of treatment and prevention. The outlet stocks the complete range of products used by physicians and nurses so there is no favoritism towards any particular manufacturer – patient welfare is the priority. Their reward for good service is your continued patronage.

The advantage of dealing with these professionals is that you can spend time discussing the products and the various aspects of treatment in a relaxed manner and at your convenience.

WOUND BED PREPARATION (DEBRIDEMENT)

This is a vital aspect of treatment designed to accelerate endogenous healing by way of preventing barriers to healing and enhancing the effectiveness of other therapeutic measures. Although it is not a new concept, it is still considered the order of the day for achieving an optimum wound bed healing surface. Debridement treatment is the activity of removing the dead tissue on top of the pressure ulcer known as the crust, scab or eschar, or simply blood clots. There are four methods of accomplishing this: a) **surgical**, where the dead tissue is removed by a scalpel or scissors; b) **mechanical**, using a range of techniques including wet-to-dry dressings, wound irrigation or whirlpool soaks; c) **enzymatic**, using various substances to biochemically clear away debris. However these products are not yet available in Canada but are available in the US.

d) **autolytic**, where certain dressings like hydrogels enhance the effectiveness of the body's own enzymes in debriding dead tissue.

Two further critical aspects of wound bed preparation include:

•Reducing bacteria burden, which can be achieved by way of debridement or by using topical antiseptics delivered through silver-based dressings or cadexomer iodine. Correcting underlying cases of poor circulation and immunosuppression may also help.
•Maintaining moisture balance, which involves the control of exudates while maintaining a moist wound environment. This is achieved through the correct use of hydrogel or absorbent dressings or through the use of mechanical devices such as topical negative pressure therapy, as described below.

Negative Pressure Wound Therapy (NPWT) – Vacuum Assisted Closure®

This uses negative pressure (a vacuum) over the wound to help promote wound healing. The leader in this field is the integrated V.A.C.® Therapy System which is a clinically proven non-invasive advanced approach to wound healing. Patented open reticulated foam dressings, Sensa T.R.A.C.® technology, and V.A.C.® work together to deliver continuous equal distribution of negative pressure across the wound area, ensure fluid is continually drawn away from the wound, helping to promote granulation tissue formation. The Integrated V.A.C.® Therapy System has been clinically proven to promote faster and more effective wound healing, improving the quality of life of patients and reducing overall therapy costs.

WARMING (THERAPEUTIC HEAT)

Traditionally, the primary objective of the application of warmth to wounds had been to relieve pain. Preoperative warming is now a standard anaesthetic practice. However, there appear to be other benefits, such as improving blood flow and oxygen tension in tissues, and reducing the risk of developing pressure ulcers; decreasing the rate of wound infection in surgery. It may also eradicate certain infections in pressure ulcers.

Warming may be applied systemically or locally. Systemic warming is usually done with specialized warming blankets

(Bair-Hugger, Arizant Health Care), or mattresses (Pegasus-Inditherm mattresses). Local warming is achieved by specially designed pads that may use an external source of electricity (Warm up dressing, Augustine Medical Inc.)

Warming is an attractive option for many reasons. It can be used prophylactically as well as therapeutically, it's simple to apply, it's inexpensive and cost effective, it may reduce the need for antibiotics and it may actually be useful in circumstances where antibiotics have failed.

ELECTRICAL STIMULATION

This is the use of an electrical current to transfer energy to a pressure ulcer or wound. There are many different waveforms available on electrotherapy equipment; the most favorable one for clinical application is HVPC (High Voltage Pulsed Current), which has been proven to be safe and effective.

Used by physical therapists for spasms and injuries, there is increasing interest in this treatment to speed up closure of chronic wounds. In one clinical study it was found that there was significant improvement in patients receiving TENS (transcutaneous electrical nerve stimulators) treatment for skin ulcers compared with patients who used a placebo (a false TENS treatment). In its clinical practice guidelines, the AHCPR recommends considering electrotherapy treatment for stages II, III and IV of pressure ulcers.

Some of the scientific explanations for its effectiveness appear related to increasing blood flow, enhancing tissue oxygenation, reducing edema, controlling infection, solubilizing blood products including necrotic tissue, and stimulating the biochemical rebuilding process. There is a wide range of optimum dose response and the relative effectiveness of different modalities of electrical stimulation.

HYPERBARIC OXYGEN

Notes

Oxygen is more than a nutrient. Most vital cellular and molecular repair processes within a pressure ulcer are directly or indirectly influenced by the available levels of oxygen. This is seen in the poor healing rates among patients with poor blood circulation and the improvement in healing when warming treatment increases the levels of tissue oxygen.

Hyperbaric oxygen is one proven method of increasing oxygen delivery to the tissues. It is achieved by patients breathing in 100% oxygen in pressurized chambers. The best way of describing how this works is to consider the process of trying to dissolve salt. When you pour a spoonful of salt into a glass of cold water, not all of the salt dissolves. Pour the same amount of salt into hot water and all the salt dissolves. What higher temperatures do for salt in water, pressure does for oxygen in the blood. At higher air pressures, more oxygen dissolves in your body.

The process involves walking into a chamber, alone or with one or more people, while you breathe oxygen through a mask or head tent. Alternatively, you may lie in a one-person chamber, the entire chamber being pressurized and filled with oxygen. It's the oxygen you breathe in, not the circulating oxygen drifting around your pressure ulcer or wound, that helps speed up healing.

For several hours after a treatment, oxygen levels remain high, encouraging capillary growth. New capillaries mean more blood gets to the site of the pressure ulcer, which can speed up healing.

This treatment should be regarded as just part of the treatment process; dressings, nutrition, infection control and other aspects of treatment should also be carried out in order for healing to take place.

OTHER PHYSICAL TREATMENTS

Magnetism, laser phototherapy, cycloidal vibration therapy and ultrasound are some of the other treatments which have been seen to have beneficial effects on various stages of the wound healing process, both in the laboratory and the clinic. Magnetism, in particular, has been shown to be effective in clinical trials. However, more controlled clinical trials with proven treatment modalities need to be documented in order for these options to be used extensively.

SKIN SUBSTITUTES

That "skin is the best dressing" is a well-known medical aphorism. The normal structural and cellular components of skin not only have a barrier function on the wound or pressure ulcer but also exert an active, positive influence on the wound environment. Tissue engineering has provided us with a number of clinically viable options to graft skin onto a wound or pressure ulcer. These products may be single layered (containing the equivalent of either epidermis or dermis) or bilayered (containing layers which mimic both the dermis and epidermis). The following are examples of skin substitutes:

Single layered products

Dermagraft®, Smith + Nephew. Newborn foreskin-derived fibroblasts when cultured on a 3-dimensional plymer scaffold remain metabolically active, producing growth factors that support wound healing. Dermagraft® is single-layered and cryopreserved.

Alloderm®, Life Cell Corporation. Cadaveric skin is processed to remove all dermal and epidermal cells, resulting in an acellular dermal collagen matrix. Following application, the graft revascularises from the wound bed and is populated by the recipient cell.

Bilayered products

Apilagraf®, Organogenesis Inc. This bioengineered bilayered skin substitute contains a dermal and epidermal layer closely resembling the architecture of the skin. It contains matrix proteins and express cytokines, but it does not contain melanocytes, langehans cells macrophages, lymphocytes, blood vessels or appendages. Apilgraf® contains neonatal foreskin fibroblasts and keratinocytes on a dermal matrix mode of pf bovine type I collagen. It has been proven to achieve faster healing in pressure ulcers.

GROWTH FACTORS

Normal wound healing is heavily dependent on a wide range of growth factors and cytokines which interact with cells and the matrix at different phases. Topical (applied to the skin) use of growth factors to speed up wound healing is theoretically promising but is still in the early days in practice.

Although not approved in Canada at the time of printing of this book, Regranex®, a PDGF (Platelet Derived Growth Factor) is the only growth factor licensed for topical use in the US. It has shown to be effective in helping heal Stage I and Stage II pressure ulcers in Stages I and II

Maggot Debridement Therapy (MDT)

Repulsive as it may sound, this treatment has proven to be effective with pressure ulcers with slough and infection and can be useful against drug resistant strains of bacteria, such as Methicillin Resistant Staphylococcus Aureus, or MRSA. Larva therapy involves the application onto the wound of necrophagous larvae of the green bottle fly (Lucilia sericata), reared in a controlled and sterile environment.

Larva therapy is cost-effective and well-tolerated. Maggots augment wound healing in the following ways:
•Having an antimicrobial effect;
•Selective debridement: secreted proteases cause rapid and selective degradation of dead tissue, and
•Larval secretions promote constructive tissue interactions at the wound site.

The limitations of this treatment are the lack of esthetic appeal and the short life of the maggots.

A LITTLE CARE GOES A LONG WAY

Well, there you have it – a complete overview of the prevention of pressure ulcers, bed sores, decubitus ulcers and wounds, as well as some general principles of treatment. Remember that pressure ulcers appear simple when they're forming but can be devastatingly serious once they've developed. It's worth making that little extra effort to guard against them.

Notes

PREVENTION & TREATMENT CHECKLIST

The risk – assessment completed and specific risk factors noted. ❏

The support people know their role and responsibilities for prevention. ❏

Patient, family members, caregiver and support staff have been comprehensively educated on pressure ulcers, especially on the causes. ❏

You have listened to the patient's feelings, concerns and understanding, especially with regard to pain and comfort issues. ❏

If the patient smokes, provide help in quitting. ❏

The skin should be inspected daily, looking for reddened areas, especially around risk areas. Do not rub reddened areas. Casts and splints should also be checked for pressure or irritation. ❏

Implement a skin care program, keeping the skin clean and dry, moisturize as necessary. ❏

The hygiene procedures are maintained and the need for incontinence pads and skin protectant considered. ❏

A turning schedule has been established. Also proper positioning and transferring techniques are used. Avoid friction and shear. ❏

Appropriate pressure redistribution devices have been obtained with special attention to the mattress and heel protectors. ❏

Understanding the wound dressing's role and how and when to change it. ❏

A nutrition plan and / or supplements are provided. Maintain hydration. ❏

An activity / exercise plan if appropriate has been established. ❏

The home layout and furniture is planned to avoid accidents ❏

A treatment plan is documented, listing supplies needed and where available, resource - contacts with phone numbers and who will assist in the home. ❏

SKIN CARE RECORD - PART 1

INSTRUCTIONS: Describe the pressure ulcer/wound using the following criteria and record in PART II of this form.

STAGES:
I – Reddened area
II – Blister or skin break
III – Skin break but exposing underneath tissue
IV – Skin break exposing actual muscle or bone

SIZE: Record size in centimeters. Use pressure ulcer measuring device if you have one.

* COLOR:
R - Red   Y - Yellow   B - Black

** DRAINAGE:
S - Serious (thin to watery)
SS - Serosanguineous (thin to red—a mixture of serum and blood)
P - Purulent (consisting of pus)

*** ODOR:
N - None   M - Mild   S - Strong

**** UNDERMINING: Separation of skin from underlying tissue.

N - None
U - Unable to determine
P - Present

***** INFLAMMATION: Record number of centimeters surrounding the pressure ulcer/wound.

CIRCLE LOCATIONS OF PRESSURE ULCERS:

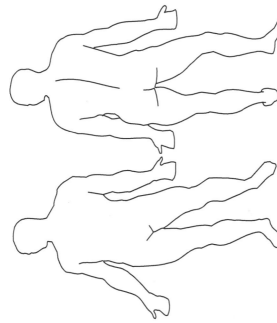

NUMBER OF ULCERS PRESENT _____

SKIN CARE RECORD - PART II

ASSESSMENT FREQUENCY: Every seven days or as changes occur in the wound/pressure ulcer.

Name:

Risk assessment score:

Date	Location	Stage	Size	Color	Drainage	Odor	Inflammation	Undermining

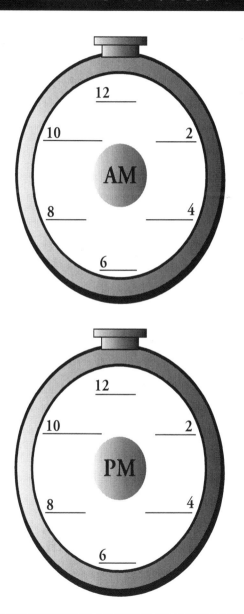

USEFUL WEBSITES

Canadian Association of Wound Care *see page 84
www.cawc.net

Canadian Association of Enterostomal Therapy
www.caet.ca

Registered Nurses Association of Ontario *see page 84
www.rnao.org

Wound Ostomy & Continence Nurses Association
www.wocn.org

National Pressure Ulcer Advisory Panel *see page 84
www.npuap.org

The Wound Healing Society
www.woundheal.org

American Academy of Wound Management
www.aawm.org

Pressure Ulcer Awareness Program
www.preventpressureulcers.com

International Wound Care Course (IIWC)
www.twhc.ca

Body1.inc
www.wounds1.com

The Wound Care information network
www.medicedu.com

Association for the advancement of wound care
www.aawc1.com

Wound Care Institute
www.woundcare.org

World Wide Wounds
www.worldwidewounds.com

European Pressure Ulcer Advisory Panel
www.epuap.org

WOUND CARE SPECIALISTS

Notes

Caring for wounds is a team effort. The patient and caregiver are the key players who can ensure a successful outcome through self care practices and compliance to the health care practitioner's treatment.

There are many different titles for health care workers and professionals involved in pressure ulcers, here is a list for your interest.

Family physician
Surgeon
Podiatrist
Chiropodist
Registered nurse
Dietician
Enterostomal nurse
Home care nurse
Physiotherapist
Occupational therapist
Plastic surgeon
Dermatologist
Pharmacist

Personal Support Workers
Home Support Workers
Unlicensed Care Providers
Home Health Aides
Home Care Aides
Nurse Aides
Nursing Assistants
Personal Support Workers
Personal Care Attendants
Unlicensed Assistive Personnel
Community Health Workers
Home care store professional

FOR MORE IN-DEPTH INFORMATION

Although this book provides comprehensive information for the layperson on pressure ulcers to achieve understanding of this health issue, there is more objective and systematic clinical information available on some of the websites listed.

If you are a health care professional, student or a reader seeking more clinical information on the subject of Pressure Ulcers, then the following authoritative website guidelines could help. The first two websites provide professional information on "best practice guidelines". These are systematically developed statements (based on best available evidence) to assist practitioners' and patients/clients' decision on appropriate health care.

Notes

The Canadian Association of Wound Care
(CAWC): www.cawc.net
Click "Resource Libarary" on the left hand side menu. Click on "clinical" from the pop up menu. Now you have two excellent resources: a) Click on the "Quick Reference Guides" topic: prevention and treatment of pressure Ulcers. This provides in summary form 12 Recommendations for Practice. For greater detail click on under, "articles"," best practices for the prevention and treatment of Pressure Ulcers". This provides 15 pages of explanation of the 12 recommendations for "best practice".

Further on this website, if you click on "education" on the left hand side menu, you will find information on a 3 – part education series which comprehensively trains you on wound care and provides a recognized qualification.

The Registered Nurses Association of Ontario
(RNAO) www.rnao.org
Click "Best Practice Guidelines" on the left hand side menu. There are 28 listed best practice guidelines choose the following: a) "Assessment and management of stage I to Stage IV pressure Ulcers". The complete guideline is a 107 page document. b) " Risk Assessment and Prevention of pressure ulcers" . This site has the complete guidelines (83 pages), a summary of the best practice guidelines and a health information fact sheet for patients.

Pressure Ulcer Awareness Program
www.preventpressureulcer.ca
This site is linked to the CAWC listed above and provides excellent information aimed at various reader categories e.g. "caring for someone", "patients", "health care professionals" etc. For the caregiver there is "Questions to ask", "prevention based on risk of patient" and "top tips for prevention"

The National Pressure Ulcer Advisory Panel
(NPUAP) www.npuap.org
This website has more detailed information on the staging of pressure ulcers as well as information on prevention of pressure ulcers. There is also a useful assessment tool called the PUSH tool.

Nutrition Guidelines Based on Stages of Pressure Ulcers*

Nutrient	Prevention	Stage I	Stage II	Stage III	Stage IV
Energy (Kcal/kg body weight)	25-35	30-35	30-35	35-40	35-40
Protein (g/kg body weight)	0.8-1.0	1-1.2	1-1.5	1-1.5 Up to 2 if needed**	1-1.5 Up to 2 If needed**
Fluids (ml/kg body weight)	30	30-35	30-35	30-35	30-35
Vitamin A	If deficiency established or suspected, 25,000 - 50,000 IU orally or 10,000 IU IV. Use for 7-10 days				
Vitamin E	15mg/day	15 mg/day	15 mg/day	15 mg/day	15 mg/day
Vitamin C	If deficiency established or suspected, 100-500 mg/day. Use for 7 days.				
Zinc	If deficiency established or suspected, 50 mg/day of elemental zinc. Use for 10 days and then re-evaluate.				
Arginine	17-24.8 g/day	17-24.8 g/day	17-24.8 g/day	17-24.8 g/day	17-24.8 g/day

- *Adapted from Dorner, B. "calculating nutritional needs for older adults." *Today's Dietitian, 2005.*
- ** Monitor renal function

Made in the USA
San Bernardino, CA
19 May 2018